48 Bodybuilder Lunch Meals High In Protein: Increase Muscle Fast Without Pills or Protein Bars

By

Joseph Correa

Certified Sports Nutritionist

COPYRIGHT

© 2015 Correa Media Group

All rights reserved

Reproduction or translation of any part of this work beyond that permitted by section 107 or 108 of the 1976 United States Copyright Act without the permission of the copyright owner is unlawful.

This publication is designed to provide accurate and authoritative information in regard to

The subject matter covered. It is sold with the understanding that neither the author nor the publisher is engaged in rendering medical advice. If medical advice or assistance is needed, consult with a doctor. This book is considered a guide and should not be used in any way detrimental to your health. Consult with a physician before starting this nutritional plan to make sure it's right for you.

ACKNOWLEDGEMENTS

The realization and success of this book could not have been possible without my family.

48 Bodybuilder Lunch Meals High In Protein: Increase Muscle Fast Without Pills or Protein Bars

By

Joseph Correa

Certified Sports Nutritionist

CONTENTS

Copyright

Acknowledgements

About The Author

Introduction

48 Bodybuilder Lunch Meals High In Protein: Increase Muscle Fast Without Pills or Protein Bars

Other Great Titles by This Author

ABOUT THE AUTHOR

As a certified sports nutritionist and professional athlete, I firmly believe that proper nutrition will help you reach your goals faster and effectively. My knowledge and experience has helped me live healthier throughout the years and which I have shared with family and friends. The more you know about eating and drinking healthier, the sooner you will want to change your life and eating habits.

Being successful in controlling your weight is important as it will improve all aspects of your life.

Nutrition is a key part in the process of getting in better shape and that's what this book is all about.

INTRODUCTION

48 Bodybuilder Lunch Meals High In Protein: Increase Muscle Fast Without Pills or Protein Bars

This book will help you increase the amount of protein you consume per day to help increase muscle mass. These meals will help increase muscle in an organized manner by adding large healthy portions of protein to your diet. Being too busy to eat right can sometimes become a problem and that's why this book will save you time and help nourish your body to achieve the goals you want. Make sure you know what you're eating by preparing it yourself or having someone prepare it for you.

This book will help you to:

-Gain muscle fast naturally.

-Improve muscle recovery.

-Have more energy.

-Naturally accelerate Your Metabolism to build more muscle.

-Improve your digestive system.

Joseph Correa is a certified sports nutritionist and a professional athlete.

48 Bodybuilder Lunch Meals High In Protein: Increase Muscle Fast Without Pills or Protein Bars

1. Chicken wraps

Ingredients:

1 pound of chicken breast, boneless and skinless

2 cups of chicken broth

1 cup of Greek yogurt

1 cup of fresh parsley, chopped

½ tsp of sea salt

¼ tsp of ground pepper

4 cups of chopped lettuce

1 cup of diced tomato

½ cup of onion, sliced

1 package of tortillas (low carb, whole wheat)

Preparation:

Combine chicken broth and chicken meat in a sauce pan over medium heat. Cover the sauce pan and allow it to boil. Cook for another 10-15 over medium-low heat. Remove from heat and drain. Let it stand for a while. Chop the meat into bite size pieces.

Meanwhile, in a large bowl, combine Greek yogurt, chicken meat, parsley, salt and pepper. Mix gently until the chicken is well coated. Spread this mixture over tortillas and top with lettuce, tomato and onion. Roll and serve.

Nutritional values for one tortilla:

Carbohydrates 14.5 g

Sugar 2.5g

Protein 21.5 g

Total fat 5g

Sodium 568.2 mg

Potassium 83.2mg

Calcium 31mg

Iron 9mg

Vitamins (vitamin A; B-6; B-12; C; D; D2; D3; K; Riboflavin; Niacin; Thiamin; K)

Calories 167

2. Italian pasta

Ingredients:

1 cup of whole grain pasta

2 cups of shrimps

1 cup of red peppers, chopped

1 tbsp of Parmesan cheese

4 tbsp of Greek yogurt

Preparation:

Use package directions to boil pasta. Drain well and let it stand.

Meanwhile, combine red peppers, Parmesan cheese and Greek yogurt in a saucepan. Let it melt over a medium temperature and add shrimps. Stir fry for 5 minutes.

Pour the shrimp sauce over pasta and serve warm.

Nutritional values per 100g:

Carbohydrates 22g

Sugar 7g

Protein 23.2 g

Total fat 6.3g

Sodium 531.5 mg

Potassium 112.1mg

Calcium 28mg

Iron 8.2mg

Vitamins (vitamin A; B-6; B-12; C; D; D2; D3; K; Riboflavin; Niacin; Thiamin; K)

Calories 212

3. Cilantro garlic burgers topped with parmesan

Ingredients:

2 cans of lentils, drained

3 cloves of garlic, minced

½ cup of breadcrumbs

¼ cup of parmesan cheese (freshly grated is best, but whatever you got will work)

1 egg, beaten

2 cups of water

½ cup of flour

salt and pepper to taste

Preparation:

In a medium size bowl, mash lentils with folk then mix with garlic, breadcrumbs and cheese. Form into patties; set aside. Whisk egg and water in bowl; flour and salt & pepper in another bowl. Coat each patty gently with flour mixture, dip into egg, then coat again with flour. Over medium-high heat in a large skillet, heat oil. Fry the burgers until lightly brown, about 2-3 minutes each side.

Serve on warm bread or in a pita with cilantro, yogurt, onion, tomatoes and whatever else you like – but this is optional!

Nutritional values per 100g:

Carbohydrates 16.1g

Sugar 4.5g

Protein 19.8g

Total fat 6.7g

Sodium 511mg

Potassium 96.1mg

Calcium 27mg

Iron 8.9mg

Vitamins (vitamin A; B-6; B-12; C; D; D2; D3; K; Riboflavin; Niacin; Thiamin; K)

Calories 195

4. Potato and cheese

Ingredients:

3 medium potatoes

½ cup of cottage cheese

¼ cup of cheddar cheese

¼ cup of organic tomato puree

¼ cup parsley, chopped

Directions

Preheat the oven to 350 degrees. Wash and peel the potatoes. Cut each potato into 2 slices and bake for 30 minutes. Remove from the oven.

Combine cottage and cheddar cheese in a bowl and spread over potato slices. Allow it to melt slightly. Top with tomato puree and chopped parsley. Serve immediately.

Nutritional values per 100g:

Carbohydrates 21.8g

Sugar 9.3g

Protein 21g

Total fat 7g

Sodium 312 mg

Potassium 61mg

Calcium 19.7mg

Iron 5mg

Vitamins (vitamin A; B-6; B-12; C; D; D2; D3; K; Riboflavin; Niacin; Thiamin; K)

Calories 154

5. Curry lentils

Ingredients:

1 cup of lentils

1 cup of low fat cream

4 cups of water

¼ tsp of salt

½ teaspoon of coriander powder

½ teaspoon of cayenne pepper

¼ tsp of turmeric powder

1 tsp of ground cumin

1 small to medium sized onion (chopped)

2 tbsp of butter

1 tbsp of chinese parsley (for garnishing)

Preparation:

Soak lentils in cool water for 1 hour to overnight, this will make the cooking process easier and less time consuming (but can be skipped). Before cooking rinse lentils and drain the excess water thoroughly.

Pour water in a large saucepan and bring to boil, then turn the heat to medium-low. In hot water add lentils, garlic, salt, coriander, pepper, and turmeric powder. Cover and leave until lentils are tender. This process will take about 30 minutes to 1 hour. You can add more water if necessary.

When lentils are soft and cooked, melt the butter in a pot over low to medium heat. Stir chopped onion until they turn golden brown, then add cumin, and fry about a minute on a low temperature. Stir constantly.

Stir the onions and butter into the lentils; cook on low heat for another 5 to 8 minutes. Add low fat cream and allow it to melt.

Garnish with chopped parsley and serve.

Nutritional values per 100g:

Carbohydrates 18.1g

Sugar 6.1g

Protein 17.5g

Total fat 3g

Sodium 112mg

Potassium 43.3mg

Calcium 19mg

Iron 6mg

Vitamins (vitamin A; B-6; B-12; C; D; D2; D3; K; Riboflavin; Niacin; Thiamin; K)

Calories 97

6. Winter chicken surprise

Ingredients:

1 pound of boneless chicken, chopped

1 2/3 cups of chicken broth

2/4 cup of chopped onions

½ cup of brown rice

½ cup of cottage cheese

3 tbsp of Greek yogurt

¼ tsp of salt

½ tsp of basil

¼ tsp of oregano

¼ tsp of thyme, crushed

1/8 tsp of garlic powder

1/8 tsp of pepper

½ cup of cheese shredded

Preparation:

Combine the chicken and onions into a skillet and cook between medium to high heat until chicken is cooked. This should take about 20-30 minutes.

Place chicken and onions into a large bowl and then add chicken broth, uncooked brown rice, basil, salt, oregano, thyme, garlic powder, pepper and cottage cheese. Mix up until everything is thoroughly combined.

Place the mixture into an ungreased 1½ quart casserole dish with a tight fitting lid.

Preheat oven to 250 degrees. Bake covered for about 30 minutes, or until rice is done, stirring it several times during cooking.

Uncover the casserole dish and top with Greek yogurt.

Bake uncovered for about five more minutes until yogurt is completely melted. Garnish with parsley before serving.

Nutritional values per 100g:

Carbohydrates 16.1g

Sugar 2.5g

Protein 23.5 g

Total fat 5g

Sodium 567.1 mg

Potassium 84.2mg

Calcium 33mg

Iron 9.4mg

Vitamins (vitamin A; B-6; B-12; C; D; D2; D3; K; Riboflavin; Niacin; Thiamin; K)

Calories 198

7. Mushroom sliders

Ingredients:

1 sweet potato

1 cup of fresh button mushrooms

1 cup of cottage cheese

3 egg whites

¾ cup of chia seeds

¾ of a cup of long grain rice

¾ of a cup of bread crumbs

1 tsp of tarragon

1 tsp of parsley

1 tsp of garlic powder

1 cup of chopped spinach

Preparation:

Pour 1 cup of water in a small saucepan. Bring it to boil and cook rice until it's slightly sticky. This should take about 10 minutes. At the same time, cook chia seeds until soft in a separate pot. Finely chop mushrooms .

Thoroughly rinse spinach. Mix all the ingredients together in a large bowl . Put the bowl into the fridge to chill for 15 to 30 minutes. Take mixture out of the fridge and form into patties. Make sure cooking surfaces are cleaned and greased before adding patties to prevent them from sticking. Fry each piece on a medium temperature for about 5 minutes on both side.

Nutritional values per 100g:

Carbohydrates 19g

Sugar 7.5g

Protein 22g

Total fat 5.8g

Sodium 532 mg

Potassium 83mg

Calcium 31.3mg

Iron 7mg

Vitamins (vitamin A; B-6; B-12; C; D; D2; D3; K; Riboflavin; Niacin; Thiamin; K)

Calories 186

8. Chia seeds – indian way

Ingredients:

1 cup of chia seeds

1 cup of low fat cream

2 cloves of garlic, chopped

1 tsp of ground ginger

¼ tsp of salt

2 small chili peppers

1 small onion, chopped

Preparation:

Use 3 cups of water and bring it to boil. Put chia seeds in it and cook it for 30 minutes on a low temperature. When tender, add spices and mix well. Cook for about 5-10 minutes on a low temperature, stirring constantly. Top with low fat cream.

Nutritional values per 100g:

Carbohydrates 12.1g

Sugar 4.5g

Protein 15 g

Total fat 4g

Sodium 263.mg

Potassium 81 mg

Calcium 11mg

Iron 3mg

Vitamins (vitamin A; B-6; B-12; C; D; D2; D3; K; Riboflavin; Niacin; Thiamin; K)

Calories 111

9. Chicken chops

Ingredients:

1 cup of chicken fillets, chopped

3 tbsp of olive oil

2 tbsp of ginger, freshly chopped

2 garlic cloves, minced

5 scallions, diced

1 tbsp of curry powder

4 carrots, chopped

4 cups of chicken broth

salt to taste

ground pepper to taste

lime

Preparation:

Heat the oil over medium heat in a saucepan. Add in and saute the garlic scallions and ginger until soft. Add in the remaining ingredients, stir and bring to boiling. Reduce the heat to low, cover and let it simmer for about 20 minutes so the meat becomes tender. Pour into bowls and serve.

Nutritional values per 100g:

Carbohydrates 13g

Sugar 5.5g

Protein 19.3 g

Total fat 4g

Sodium 363.2 mg

Potassium 82.1mg

Calcium 21mg

Iron 4.3mg

Vitamins (vitamin A; B-6; B-12; C; D; D2; D3; K; Riboflavin; Niacin; Thiamin; K)

Calories 134

10. Lentil burgers

Ingredients:

1 clove of garlic, peeled

½ tsp salt

1 cup of chopped walnuts

¼ tsp of black pepper, finely grounded

2 cups of rinsed lentils

2 tsp of canola oil

2 pieces of wheat bread torn into bite sized pieces

4 wheat burger buns

1 cup of chopped lettuce, red onions and tomatoes

Preparation:

Chop up the garlic clove as finely as possible. Add in the other spices (salt and pepper) to the garlic mash and mix well. Next put the nuts into a food processor and finely chop them as well before adding them to the garlic mash. Add the pieces of bread next and then finally, the lentils. Mix well, either by hand or food processor (I recommend the food processor) until the mass of ingredients come together in a mass. Remove mix and patty out four burgers from it. You are now ready to cook these beauties! Heat up the oil in a skillet set on medium heat. Add the patties and cook until each one is nicely browned on both sides.This should take no more than six minutes to complete.Put those patties on a bun, add the fixings and you have yourself a delicious and healthy protein lunch!

Nutritional values per 100g:

Carbohydrates 25g

Sugar 13.2g

Protein 26.3 g

Total fat 11g

Sodium 575 mg

Potassium 92mg

Calcium 28mg

Iron 9.7mg

Vitamins (vitamin A; B-6; B-12; C; D; D2; D3; K; Riboflavin; Niacin; Thiamin; K)

Calories 194

11. Chickpea & chili soup

Ingredients:

2 tsp of cumin seeds

½ cup of chili flakes

½ cup of lentils

1 tbsp of olive oil

1 red onion , chopped

3 cups of vegetable stock

1 cup of can tomatoes, whole or chopped

½ cup of chickpeas

small bunch of coriander, roughly chopped

4 tbsp of Greek yogurt, for serving

Preparation:

Heat a large saucepan and dry-fry the cumin seeds and chili flakes for 1 minute or until they start to jump around the pan and release their aromas. Add the oil and onion, and cook for 5 minutes. Stir in the lentils, stock and tomatoes, then bring to the boil. Simmer for 15 minutes until the lentils have softened.

Mix the soup with a stick blender or in a food processor until it is a rough purée, pour back into the pan and add the chickpeas. Heat gently, season well and stir in the coriander. Finish with a dollop of yogurt and coriander leaves.

Nutritional values per 100g:

Carbohydrates 18g

Sugar 9.8g

Protein 21g

Total fat 7g

Sodium 529mg

Potassium 63.1mg

Calcium 21mg

Iron 8.9mg

Vitamins (vitamin A; B-6; B-12; C; D; D2; D3; K; Riboflavin; Niacin; Thiamin; K)

Calories 120

12. Quinoa & Shrimp Paella

Ingredients:

1 pound of frozen shrimps, cleaned

1 cup of dry quinoa

2 cups of chicken broth

1 medium onion, diced

2 cloves of garlic, minced

1 tbsp of olive oil

1 bay leaf

½ tsp of red pepper, ground

½ tsp of green pepper, ground

½ tsp of black pepper, ground

¼ tsp of sea salt

½ cup of chopped dry tomatoes

1 cup of green peas

1 tsp of organic seafood seasoning

Preparation:

Use package instructions to prepare quinoa. Meanwhile, wash and drain shrimps. Sprinkle them with a pinch of salt and leave in the refrigerator.

In a large saucepan, heat the olive oil over a medium temperature. Add onions and stir well. Fry for about 5 minutes. Add garlic and saute for 1 minute. Now add quinoa, chicken broth and spices. Cover and allow it to boil. Reduce heat and continue cooking for another 10-15 minutes. You don't want any liquid left.

Remove from heat and add dry tomatoes, peas and shrimps. Cover and allow it to stand for about 5 minutes before serving.

Nutritional values per 1 cup:

Carbohydrates 31g

Sugar 3.8g

Protein 27g

Total fat 6g

Sodium 412mg

Potassium 623mg

Calcium 171.7mg

Iron 0.83mg

Vitamins (Vitamin C total ascorbic acid; B-6; B-12; Folate-DFE; A-RAE; A-IU; E-alpha-tocopherol; D; D-D2+D3; Thianin; Niacin)

Calories 283

13. British chia seeds

Ingredients:

2 cups of chia seeds

2 tbs Worcestershire Sauce

1 tsp Malt vinegar

2 tsp of salt

2 cups of water

Preparation:

It is best to soak the seeds for 8-12 hours, but if you can't then cook them in water for 35 - 45 minutes until they start to soften.

When chia seeds start to soften, add other ingredients. Cook until seeds are soft enough that they will mash easily with a large spoon.

Make sure there is a small amount of liquid in the mixture until the very end of the cooking process. It's best to add half a cup of water at a time and stir frequently.

Nutritional values per 100g:

Carbohydrates 12g

Sugar 2 g

Protein 11g

Total fat 3.4g

Sodium 166.9 mg

Potassium 73.1mg

Calcium 21mg

Iron 5.1mg

Vitamins (vitamin A; B-6; B-12; C; D; D2; D3; K; Riboflavin; Niacin; Thiamin; K)

Calories 146

14. Barbecue peas

Ingredients:

2 cups of canned peas, washed and rinsed

5 cups of water

½ cup of non fat yogurt

½ cup of Greek yogurt

2 tbsp of brown sugar

1 tbsp of vinegar

1 tsp of mustard

1 tsp of Worcestershire sauce

2 tsp of tomato sauce

1 small chopped onion

Preparation:

Preheat your oven at 350 degrees. Pour peas in water, and bring it to boil. Let it boil for 30 minutes, or until tender. Make sure that they remain whole. Add all the ingredients to the boiled and tender peas, and stir the mixture to combine them well. Pour the peas in a baking dish an and bake for 45 minutes. Top with Greek yogurt.

Nutritional values per 100g:

Carbohydrates 22.3g

Sugar 6.1g

Protein 23.1 g

Total fat 6g

Sodium 428.1 mg

Potassium 73.2mg

Calcium 33mg

Iron 5mg

Vitamins (vitamin A; B-6; B-12; C; D; D2; D3; K; Riboflavin; Niacin; Thiamin; K)

Calories 167.5

15. Buckwheat pasta with mozzarella

Ingredients:

1 small pack of buckwheat pasta

½ cup of chia seeds powder

1 small can of sugar-free tomato sauce

1 small mozzarella

1 tsp of rosemary

olive oil

salt

Preparation:

Use package instructions to cook pasta. Wash it and drain. Chop mozzarella into small pieces and mix with tomato sauce. Add chia seeds powder to this mixture. Cook this sauce for about 10 minutes, stirring constantly. Add rosemary, olive oil and salt. Cook for another 4-5 minutes and pour over pasta.

Nutritional values per 100g:

Carbohydrates 20.1g

Sugar 8.5g

Protein 21.3 g

Total fat 7g

Sodium 268mg

Potassium 73.3mg

Calcium 22mg

Iron 5mg

Vitamins (vitamin A; B-6; B-12; C; D; D2; D3; K; Riboflavin; Niacin; Thiamin; K)

Calories 160

16. Turkey with vegetables

Ingredients:

1 pound of turkey, skinless and boneless

1 bunch of spinach

1 cup of chopped broccoli

¼ tsp of sea salt

¼ tsp of red pepper

Preparation:

Wash and cut turkey into bite size pieces. Put it in a large saucepan and add water to cover the meat. Bring it to boil over a high temperature. Cook until the meat is tender. Reduce the heat, add spinach and broccoli. Stir well and cook for another 15 minutes on a very low temperature. Add spices and serve warm.

Nutritional values per 100g:

Carbohydrates 10g

Sugar 2.4g

Protein 17.5 g

Total fat 4.8g

Sodium 161.4 mg

Potassium 31.5mg

Calcium 11mg

Iron 5.9mg

Vitamins (vitamin A; B-6; B-12; C; D; D2; D3; K; Riboflavin; Niacin; Thiamin; K)

Calories 112

17. Spinach ravioli

Ingredients:

3 cups of whole grain flour

2 cups of water

3 eggs

3 egg whites

6 tablespoons of olive oil

2 cups of spinach, chopped

1 cup of cottage cheese

1 cup of low fat yogurt

¼ tsp of salt

¼ tsp of pepper

Preparation:

In a large bowl, combine flour, water, eggs, egg whites, olive oil and a pinch of salt. You want to make a smooth dough. Cover and let it stand in a warm place for about 30 minutes.

Briefly boil spinach in salted water, drain and cut. Combine with cottage cheese, yogurt, salt and pepper.

Roll the dough thinly, cut out circles using molds and put in each hemisphere spoon of stuffing. Replace the second part of dough and press the edges with a fork so that the stuffing does not fall off.

Cook ravioli in boiling water to which you have added a little salt and olive oil. It should take about 15 minutes. Remove from the saucepan, drain and serve.

Nutritional values per 100g:

Carbohydrates 21.7g

Sugar 9.5g

Protein 28 g

Total fat 5g

Sodium 571.3 mg

Potassium 92.3mg

Calcium 40mg

Iron 9.8mg

Vitamins (vitamin A; B-6; B-12; C; D; D2; D3; K; Riboflavin; Niacin; Thiamin; K)

Calories 181

18. Grilled veal steak with fresh vegetables

Ingredients:

1 thick steak

1 medium carrot

1 bunch of lettuce

1 small tomato

1 small onion

2 tsp of Greek yogurt

1 cup of low fat cream

2 pickles

¼ tsp of salt

1/8 tsp of pepper

2 tbsp of olive oil

Preparation:

Wash and pat dry the steak with a kitchen paper. Cut into bite sizes and set aside. Heat up the olive oil over a medium temperature and fry the meat for about 15 minutes, stirring constantly. Remove from the heat and let it stand.

Wash and cut vegetables into small pieces. Combine with Greek yogurt and low fat cream. Season with salt and pepper and add meat in it.

Serve cold.

Nutritional values per 100g:

Carbohydrates 22.3g

Sugar 6.2g

Protein 23 g

Total fat 7g

Sodium 382.6 mg

Potassium 52mg

Calcium 21mg

Iron 5mg

Vitamins (vitamin A; B-6; B-12; C; D; D2; D3; K; Riboflavin; Niacin; Thiamin; K)

Calories 175

19. Grilled salmon

Ingredients:

4 thick salmon fillets

2 tbsp of fresh lemon juice

¼ cup of fresh orange juice

¼ cup of low fat cream sauce

½ cup of chopped onions

1 tsp of dried parsley

1 tsp of ground garlic

cooking spray

Preparation:

In a large bowl, combine lemon juice, orange juice, low fat cream sauce, onions, parsley and garlic. Mix well to make a marinade. Add salmon fillets. Cover a bowl with a tight lid and leave in the refrigerator for about an hour.

Prepare a grill pan and sprinkle with cooking spray. Heat up over a high temperature and add salmon fillets. Fry for about 5 minutes on each side. You can add some more marinade while frying. Serve immediately.

Nutritional values per 100g:

Carbohydrates 17.2g

Sugar 3.5g

Protein 21.5 g

Total fat 5g

Sodium 528.1 mg

Potassium 84.1mg

Calcium 30mg

Iron 9mg

Vitamins (vitamin A; B-6; B-12; C; D; D2; D3; K; Riboflavin; Niacin; Thiamin; K)

Calories 171

20. Bean and mushroom mix

Ingredients:

2 cups of button mushrooms, sliced

1 cup of canned green beans, cooked

½ cup of onions, chopped

1 tbsp of fresh celery, chopped

¼ cup of apple vinegar

4 tbsp of sea salt

5 tbsp of extra virgin olive oil

1/3 cup of toasted almonds

1/3 cup of sliced dried figs

Preparation:

In a medium sized bowl, combine the onions with apple vinegar and let it stand for about 10-15 minutes. Add salt and 2 tbsp of olive oil.

Meanwhile, heat up the olive oil in a large saucepan and add the mushrooms. Cook for few minutes, stirring constantly. Remove from the heat when the mushrooms release their water. Add the beans, celery, figs and almonds to the saucepan. Mix well with mushrooms. Fry for several more minutes and remove from heat.

Pour the onion marinade on top and serve.

Nutritional values per 100g:

Carbohydrates 22.7g

Sugar 7.1g

Protein 19g

Total fat 7.4g

Sodium 570 mg

Potassium 71.2mg

Calcium 35.3mg

Iron 8mg

Vitamins (vitamin A; B-6; B-12; C; D; D2; D3; K; Riboflavin; Niacin; Thiamin; K)

Calories 167

21. Roasted lentils:

Ingredients:

½ cups of uncooked lentils

1 tbsp of salt

2 tbsp of olive oil

1 tsp of pepper

1 tsp of red chili powder

1 tsp of cinnamon powder

Preparation:

First you want to cook lentils. Pour about 2 cups of water in a saucepan and bring it to boil. Add lentils and boil for about 15-20 minutes, until soft from inside and still hold their shape. Remove from the heat and rinse well with cold water. Drain your chia seeds and set aside.

Preheat the oven to 300 degrees. In a large bowl, coat the lentils with salt, olive oil, pepper, red chili powder and cinnamon. Spread the lentils over a medium sized baking dish and bake for about 20 minutes.

Prepared like this, lentils can be stored in the air-tight container for about 15 days.

Nutritional values per 100g:

Carbohydrates 19g

Sugar 7.5g

Protein 17 g

Total fat 4.3g

Sodium 188mg

Potassium 72 mg

Calcium 27mg

Iron 5.9mg

Vitamins (vitamin A; B-6; B-12; C; D; D2; D3; K; Riboflavin; Niacin; Thiamin; K)

Calories 123

22. Chia seeds with curry & fresh lime

Ingredients:

3 tsp of vegetable oil

2 tbsp of ginger, freshly grated

2 cloves of garlic, minced

3 carrots, chopped

1 large potato, chopped

1 small onion, chopped

1 cup of dry chia seeds

4 cups of chicken broth

1 tsp of curry powder

¾ tsp of salt

¼ tsp of pepper

lime wedges for serving

Preparation:

Heat oil in large saucepan over medium heat. Add the ginger, garlic, chopped carrots, potatoes, and onions.

Saute' until vegetables become soft. Add the chia seeds, broth, and seasonings, stirring well while turning up the heat to medium high until mixture comes to a boil. Cover, turn heat back down to medium-low and simmer for 15 to 20 minutes, stirring occasionally, until seeds are tender and most of the liquid is absorbed. Serve with fresh lime wedges.

Nutritional values per 100g:

Carbohydrates 27g

Sugar 11g

Protein 26.7 g

Total fat 8g

Sodium 598 mg

Potassium 92.1mg

Calcium 41mg

Iron 11mg

Vitamins (vitamin A; B-6; B-12; C; D; D2; D3; K; Riboflavin; Niacin; Thiamin; K)

Calories 182

23. Fresh legumes – mexican way

Ingredients:

1 ½ cups of fresh legumes, chopped

1 ½ tbs of red chili powder or one tbs of Cayenne pepper

1 ½ tbs of onion flakes or 1 tbs of onion powder

¾ tsp of oregano

¾ tsp of garlic powder

¾ tsp of ground cumin

¾ tsp of salt

3 cups of water to start (add more throughout the cooking process)

Preparation:

It is best to soak the legumes the night before. Wash them in a colander and then put them in a saucepan and cover them with plenty of water and let soak for 24 hours. Then drain the legumes. In a large skillet, spread the legumes out and add three cups of water. Add the recipe spices and cook over a medium heat until legumes are soft enough that they can be mashed. You will need to add more water during the cooking process as your legumes will continue to absorb it. Add water a half-cup at a time, just enough to keep the mixture moist with some visible liquid. The entire cooking process will take about 45 minutes. Legumes will be soft to chew. Mash after cooking if preferred.

Nutritional values per 100g:

Carbohydrates 17.1g

Sugar 3.5g

Protein 20.5 g

Total fat 5g

Sodium 568mg

Potassium 81.2mg

Calcium 30mg

Iron 5.1mg

Vitamins (vitamin A; B-6; B-12; C; D; D2; D3; K; Riboflavin; Niacin; Thiamin; K)

Calories 177

24. Lemon shrimps

Ingredients:

1 pound of large shrimps, peeled

2 tbsp of lemon juice

2 fresh lemons, cut into thin slices

5 tbsp of olive oil

½ tsp of sea salt

½ tsp of red pepper, ground

½ tsp of black pepper, ground

1 tbsp of garlic, minced

10 bey leaves

Preparation:

Wash and drain your shrimps. In a large bowl combine lemon juice, 3 tbsp of olive oil, sea salt, black and red pepper, bey leaves and garlic to make a marinade. Soak the shrimps in it. Cover the bowl and leave in the refrigerator for about 10 minutes.

Heat up 2 tbsp of olive oil over a high temperature in a grill saucepan. Fry shrimps for about 15 minutes, stirring constantly. If necessary, add some marinade while frying.

Decorate with lemon slices and serve.

Nutritional values per 100g:

Carbohydrates 11g

Sugar 6.5g

Protein 17.1 g

Total fat 6g

Sodium 232.1 mg

Potassium 53.1mg

Calcium 32mg

Iron 4mg

Vitamins (vitamin A; B-6; B-12; C; D; D2; D3; K; Riboflavin; Niacin; Thiamin; K)

Calories 124

25. Nacho casserole

Ingredients:

1 pound of ground beef

1 small onion, peeled and chopped

1 cup of spicy red beans

½ cup of canned corn, cooked

½ cup of sugar-free tomato sauce

2 tbsp of taco seasoning mix

1 cup of cottage cheese

1 cup of chopped green onions

Preparation:

Cook ground beef over a medium-high temperature, stirring occasionally. This process should take about 30 minutes. Remove from heat and drain well. Cut into bite size pieces and combine with red beans, corn, tomato sauce and seasoning mix. Stir well and simmer over medium heat for about 10 minutes.

Preheat oven to 350 degrees. Pour half of this mixture into baking casserole pan. Top with cottage cheese and green onions and add the remaining beef mixture. Bake for about 25 minutes.

Nutritional values per 100g:

Carbohydrates 27g

Sugar 6.5g

Protein 29.5 g

Total fat 11g

Sodium 611 mg

Potassium 72mg

Calcium 27mg

Iron 6.7mg

Vitamins (vitamin A; B-6; B-12; C; D; D2; D3; K; Riboflavin; Niacin; Thiamin; K)

Calories 198

26. Striped bass

Ingredients:

4 large striped bass

1 tablespoon olive oil

½ tsp of sea salt

¼ tsp of black pepper

1 cup cottage cheese

Preparation:

Combine oil salt and pepper. Use a kitchen brush to spread this mixture over fish. Grill fish over a medium-high temperature, on each side for about 5 minutes. Serve with cottage cheese.

Nutritional values per 100g:

Carbohydrates 9.8g

Sugar 2.5g

Protein 24 g

Total fat 3g

Sodium 112 mg

Potassium 24mg

Calcium 12mg

Iron 2.3mg

Vitamins (vitamin A; B-6; B-12; C; D; D2; D3; K; Riboflavin; Niacin; Thiamin; K)

Calories 143

27. Chicken mix

Ingredients:

2 large chicken fillets, boneless

1 medium tomato, peeled and chopped

1 carrot, peeled and grated

1 onion, peeled and chopped

3 tbsp of olive oil

3 tbsp of sour cream

¼ tsp of salt

Preparation:

Wash and pat dry the meat. Cut into bite size pieces. Heat up the olive oil in a saucepan over a medium-high temperature. Add meat and fry for about 15 minutes, stirring occasionally.

Meanwhile, peel and cut the vegetables into small pieces. Add to the saucepan and mix well with meat. Fry over a low temperature for another 10 minutes, or until all the liquid evaporates. Remove from the saucepan. Add sour cream and salt. Serve warm.

Nutritional values per 100g:

Carbohydrates 24g

Sugar 11.5g

Protein 29.5 g

Total fat 10g

Sodium 462.1 mg

Potassium 63.1mg

Calcium 11mg

Iron 5.6mg

Vitamins (vitamin A; B-6; B-12; C; D; D2; D3; K; Riboflavin; Niacin; Thiamin; K)

Calories 165

28. Steak salad

Ingredients:

1 thin steak

5 lettuce leaves

1 tsp of chopped radicchio

2-3 arugula leaves

4 tbsp of olive oil

3 lemon slices

1 tomato

¼ cup of ground walnuts

½ cup of cottage cheese

¼ tsp of salt

Preparation:

Wash and pat dry the steak. Heat up the olive oil over a medium temperature and fry the meat for about 10 minutes on each side, or until tender. Remove from pan and soak the excess oil with kitchen paper.Cut it into cubes and set aside.

Wash and cut the vegetables in a large bowl. Add the meat, ground walnuts and cottage cheese. Season with salt and decorate with lemon slices before serving.

Nutritional values per 100g:

Carbohydrates 29g

Sugar 14.2g

Protein 31 g

Total fat 13g

Sodium 602 mg

Potassium 97mg

Calcium 33mg

Iron 11mg

Vitamins (vitamin A; B-6; B-12; C; D; D2; D3; K; Riboflavin; Niacin; Thiamin; K)

Calories 202

29. Seafood - Mediterranean way

Ingredients:

1 small pack of frozen mixed seafood

1 tbsp of olive oil

1 small onion

1 cup of cherry tomatoes

1 tsp of chopped, dry rosemary

¼ tsp of salt

1 tbsp of freshly squeezed lemon juice

Preparation

Heat up the olive oil in a saucepan. Fry frozen seafood for about 15 minutes, over a medium temperature (try the octopus, it takes the most time to tender). You can add some water if necessary – about ¼ of cup will be enough. Stir occasionally. Remove from frying pan and allow it to cool for about an hour.

Meanwhile chop the vegetables into very small pieces. In a large bowl, combine the vegetables with seafood and season with salt, rosemary and lemon juice.

Serve cold.

Nutritional values per 100g:

Carbohydrates 18.3g

Sugar 5.5g

Protein 20.5 g

Total fat 3.4g

Sodium 390.2 mg

Potassium 53mg

Calcium 22mg

Iron 7mg

Vitamins (vitamin A; B-6; B-12; C; D; D2; D3; K; Riboflavin; Niacin; Thiamin; K)

Calories 114

30. Grilled sea bream

Ingredients:

1 fresh sea bream, scaled and gutted

1 bunch of fresh parsley, finely chopped

¼ cup of freshly squeezed lemon juice

4 tbsp of olive oil

¼ tsp of sea salt

Preparation:

Wash the fish, and using your hands soak the fish in lemon juice and olive oil. Grill it over a medium heat for about 15-20 minutes, until nice golden brown color. Remove from the heat and sprinkle with fresh parsley. Serve immediately.

Nutritional values per 100g:

Carbohydrates 10.g

Sugar 2.5g

Protein 23.5 g

Total fat 11g

Sodium 534.2 mg

Potassium 81.2mg

Calcium 32mg

Iron 7mg

Vitamins (vitamin A; B-6; B-12; C; D; D2; D3; K; Riboflavin; Niacin; Thiamin; K)

Calories 170

31. Fried tuna steak

Ingredients:

4 pieces of tuna steak (about 1 ounce each)

¼ cup of lemon juice

1 tsp of sea salt

½ tsp of red pepper

2 tbsp of chopped parsley

2 tbsp of chopped rosemary

6 tbsp olive oil

6 cloves of garlic, chopped

Preparation:

In a large bowl, mix the lemon juice, 2 tbsp of olive oil, sea salt, red pepper, chopped parsley and chopped rosemary. Combine all the ingredients to get a smooth marinade. Place the tuna steaks in this marinade and cover with a tight lid. Let it stand in the refrigerator for about an hour.

Preheat 4 tbsp of olive oil over a high heat. Fry tuna steaks for 5-6 minutes on each side. Remove from the saucepan and serve.

Nutritional values per 100g:

Carbohydrates 16.1g

Sugar 8.5g

Protein 24.1 g

Total fat 5.3g

Sodium 511.1 mg

Potassium 82.1mg

Calcium 23mg

Iron 4mg

Vitamins (vitamin A; B-6; B-12; C; D; D2; D3; K; Riboflavin; Niacin; Thiamin; K)

Calories 151

32. Lemon calamari

Ingredients:

8 large calamari tubes

¼ cup of lemon juice

3 cloves of garlic, chopped

1 tbsp of chopped rosemary

5 tbsp of olive oil

1 tsp of sea salt

¼ tsp of pepper

1 tbsp of fresh lemon zest

Few fresh parsley leaves

Preparation:

Combine the lemon juice, garlic, chopped rosemary, sea salt, pepper and lemon zest in a bowl. Fill the calamari tubes with this mixture. Let it stand for about an hour. Preheat the olive oil over a high temperature. Place the calamari in a saucepan and fry for 5 minutes on each side. Decorate with some fresh parsley leaves before serving.

Nutritional values per 100g:

Carbohydrates 18g

Sugar 7.5g

Protein 20 g

Total fat 6g

Sodium 462.1 mg

Potassium 53.2mg

Calcium 30mg

Iron 9.6mg

Vitamins (vitamin A; B-6; B-12; C; D; D2; D3; K; Riboflavin; Niacin; Thiamin; K)

Calories 127

33. Grilled beef with almonds

Ingredients:

3 large beef steaks

1 large onion, cut into thin slices

4 cups of baby spinach, chopped

1 tsp of garlic, chopped

½ tsp of ginger, minced

¼ cup of lemon juice

¼ cup of almonds

1 tbsp of lime juice

2 tbsp of water

1 tbsp of organic fish sauce, sugar-free

4 tbsp of vegetable oil

Cooking Instructions

Wash and pat dry the beef steaks. Cut into bite size pieces and set aside.

Peel the onion and cut into thin slices. Heat up the vegetable oil over a medium heat and fry the onions until gold brown color. Add chopped baby spinach and garlic. Mix well and fry for about 5 minutes, until the water from the spinach evaporates. Stir well and remove from the heat.

In a large bowl combine the baby spinach with ginger, lemon juice, water, almonds and fish sauce. Mix well with a fork. Soak the beef steak pieces in it and return to saucepan. Add some more water if necessary. Cook over a low temperature for about 30 minutes, stirring occasionally.

When the water evaporates, remove from the heat and add lime juice. Allow it to cool for about 20-30 minutes and serve.

Nutritional values per 100g:

Carbohydrates 29.1g

Sugar 16.1g

Protein 33 g

Total fat 12g

Sodium 521.4 mg

Potassium 84.1mg

Calcium 21mg

Iron 8mg

Vitamins (vitamin A; B-6; B-12; C; D; D2; D3; K; Riboflavin; Niacin; Thiamin; K)

Calories 243

34. Green chicken

Ingredients:

3 pieces of chicken breast (about 1 pound)

2 cups of spinach, chopped

1 cup of low fat yogurt

3 green peppers

3 chili peppers

2 small onions, chopped

1 tbsp of ground ginger

1 tsp of red pepper powder

4 tbsp of oil

salt to taste

Preparation:

Wash and pat dry the chicken using a kitchen paper. Chop into bite size pieces. Finely chop onion and peppers and set aside.

Heat up the oil in a large weasel. Add onions and peppers and sauté for few minutes. Now add chicken breast pieces, ground ginger, red pepper powder and salt. Stir-fry for ten minutes, or until the chicken turns light brown.

Meanwhile, combine low fat yogurt with spinach in a food processor. Mix well for 30 seconds. Add this mixture to the weasel and fry until the spinach gets well mashed. Cover the weasel, remove from the heat and let it stand for about 10 minutes before serving.

Nutritional values per 100g:

Carbohydrates 21g

Sugar 7.2g

Protein 25.1 g

Total fat 7g

Sodium 668.2 mg

Potassium 73.7mg

Calcium 22mg

Iron 8mg

Vitamins (vitamin A; B-6; B-12; C; D; D2; D3; K; Riboflavin; Niacin; Thiamin; K)

Calories 173

35. Coconut cubes

Ingredients:

3 large pieces of chicken breast, skinless, boneless

1 cup of coconut flakes, unsweetened

½ cup of rice flour

1 large egg

2 egg whites

1 cup of almond milk

¼ tsp of ground red pepper

3 tbsp of coconut oil

Preparation:

Wash and pat dry chicken meat. Cut into 1 inch thick strips. Sprinkle with pepper and place in a large bowl. Add rice flour, almond milk, egg and egg whites and stir well. Dredge chicken in this mixture. Add coconut and shake off the excess mixture.

Heat up the coconut oil over a medium temperature. Fry your chicken strips for about 10 minutes. Remove from the saucepan and serve.

Nutritional values per 100g:

Carbohydrates 26g

Sugar 9.5g

Protein 31.5 g

Total fat 11g

Sodium 598.1 mg

Potassium 93.2mg

Calcium 21mg

Iron 7.8mg

Vitamins (vitamin A; B-6; B-12; C; D; D2; D3; K; Riboflavin; Niacin; Thiamin; K)

Calories 197

36. Turkey thighs in garlic

Ingredients:

10 medium turkey thighs

1 cup of turkey broth

2 medium onions, chopped

2 cloves of garlic, ground

3 small chili peppers, chopped

¼ tsp of sea salt

¼ tsp of black pepper, ground

1 tsp of dried oregano

¾ cup of rice flower

1 cup of brown rice

3 tbsp of olive oil

Preparation:

Wash and drain turkey thighs. Set aside.

Combine salt, pepper and oregano in a small bowl. Sprinkle over turkey. Dredge turkey thighs in the rice flour. Heat up the olive oil over a medium temperature and fry turkey for about 5 minutes on each side. Remove from the saucepan. Add the onions and garlic to the same pot and fry for about 5 minutes, stirring constantly. Add turkey broth and bring it to boil. Add rice and chili peppers and cook for about 10-15 minutes. Remove from the heat. Add turkey thighs, cover and let it stand for about 30 minutes before serving.

Nutritional values per 100g:

Carbohydrates 19.1g

Sugar 5.5g

Protein 23.5 g

Total fat 5g

Sodium 538.7 mg

Potassium 85.2mg

Calcium 32mg

Iron 9.9mg

Vitamins (vitamin A; B-6; B-12; C; D; D2; D3; K; Riboflavin; Niacin; Thiamin; K)

Calories 147

37. Chicken in mushroom sauce

Ingredients:

1 pound of chicken meat, skinless

2 tbsp of all purpose flour

1 cup of button mushrooms

1 cup of green beans, cooked

¼ cup of chicken broth

½ tsp of sea salt

¼ tsp of black pepper

4 tbsp of olive oil

Preparation:

Wash and pat dry the chicken meat. In a large bowl, combine all purpose flour with salt and pepper. Coat the chicken with the flour and set aside. Heat up the olive oil over a medium temperature and fry chicken meat for about 5 minutes on each side. Remove from the saucepan and transfer to a plate. In the same saucepan add chicken broth, green beans and button mushrooms. Bring it to boil and cook for 2-3 minutes. Return the chicken and cook for another 20 minutes, stirring occasionally, until the water evaporates. Serve warm.

Nutritional values per 100g:

Carbohydrates 15 g

Sugar 2.5g

Protein 27.5 g

Total fat 11g

Sodium 531.1 mg

Potassium 82.1mg

Calcium 11mg

Iron 5mg

Vitamins (vitamin A; B-6; B-12; C; D; D2; D3; K; Riboflavin; Niacin; Thiamin; K)

Calories 136

38. Black beans with eggs

Ingredients:

1 cup of canned black beans, cooked

4 eggs

½ cup of cottage cheese

½ cup of tomato sauce, sugar free

½ cup of avocado, chopped

1 tsp of fresh lemon juice

3 tbsp of coconut oil

½ tsp of oregano

Preparation:

Preheat the oven to 350 degrees. In a large bowl, combine the ingredients and mix well. Place the mixture in a medium casserole baking dish. Bake until crisp, for about 10 minutes. Remove from the oven, cut into 4 equal pieces and serve.

Nutritional values per 100g:

Carbohydrates 22 g

Sugar 6.5g

Protein 26.5 g

Total fat 11g

Sodium 468 mg

Potassium 82.1mg

Calcium 20mg

Iron 6.5mg

Vitamins (vitamin A; B-6; B-12; C; D; D2; D3; K; Riboflavin; Niacin; Thiamin; K)

Calories 181

39. Pan roasted lamb

Ingredients:

3 pounds of chopped lamb cutlets, boneless

1 cup of lentils

5 tbsp of olive oil

½ cup of lemon juice

5 cloves of garlic, minced

1 tsp of sea salt

½ tsp of ground pepper

Preparation:

Wash and cut cutlets into bite size cubes. Set aside.

Preheat the oven to 350 degrees. Grease the baking dish with 1 tbsp of olive oil and put the meat in it.

In a large bowl, combine remaining olive oil with lemon juice, garlic, salt and pepper. Using a spoon, arrange the lentils along the inside edge of the baking dish. Pour the lemon juice mixture over the meat and lentils.

Bake for about 50 minutes and serve warm.

Nutritional values per 100g:

Carbohydrates 16g

Sugar 7.5g

Protein 26.5 g

Total fat 10g

Sodium 531.2 mg

Potassium 63.1mg

Calcium 31mg

Iron 6mg

Vitamins (vitamin A; B-6; B-12; C; D; D2; D3; K; Riboflavin; Niacin; Thiamin; K)

Calories 201

40. Crispy salmon slices

Ingredients:

6 thick salmon slices

1 cup of almond milk

3 large eggs

1 tsp of garlic powder

½ tsp of red pepper, ground

½ tsp of sea salt

1 cup of Greek yogurt

2 tbsp of canola oil

Preparation:

Combine the almond milk, eggs, garlic powder, red pepper, salt and Greek yogurt in a bowl. Place salmon slices in it, cover and marinate for about an hour.

Preheat the oven to 350 degrees. Pour the almond slices along with marinade in a small baking dish. Bake for 35 minutes. Remove from the oven, cut into 4 equal pieces and serve warm.

Nutritional values per 100g:

Carbohydrates 19.2g

Sugar 7.5g

Protein 29.5 g

Total fat 11g

Sodium 531 mg

Potassium 63mg

Calcium 31.2mg

Iron 9.1mg

Vitamins (vitamin A; B-6; B-12; C; D; D2; D3; K; Riboflavin; Niacin; Thiamin; K)

Calories 177

41. Chicken chops

Ingredients:

1 pound of chicken breast, boneless

1 large cucumber, peeled and sliced

1 medium onion, peeled and chopped

1 tsp of salt

2 tbsp of olive oil

2 tbsp of fresh lemon juice

1 tsp of ground chili pepper

1 cup of Greek yogurt

Preparation:

Wash and chop the chicken meat. Pat dry with kitchen paper. Heat up the olive oil over a high temperature. Add chopped onion and fry for about 10 minutes, or until golden brown. Stir constantly. Now you can add chicken chops and cucumber. Mix well and fry over a medium temperature for about 15 minutes. Meanwhile, combine Greek yogurt with chili pepper, lemon juice and salt. Add to saucepan and mix well with chicken. Cover and let it stand for about 10 minutes. Remove from the heat and serve.

Nutritional values per 100g:

Carbohydrates 16g

Sugar 3.5g

Protein 20.5 g

Total fat 5.7g

Sodium 518.1 mg

Potassium 83.1mg

Calcium 31.4mg

Iron 7mg

Vitamins (vitamin A; B-6; B-12; C; D; D2; D3; K; Riboflavin; Niacin; Thiamin; K)

Calories 160

42. Red beans mix

Ingredients:

1 cup of red beans, canned and cooked

½ cup of green beans

½ cup of button mushrooms

1 cup of cottage cheese

1 cup of Greek yogurt

2 egg whites

2 tbsp of coconut oil

1 tsp of sea salt

Preparation:

Combine the ingredients in a food processor. Mix well for 30 seconds. Preheat the oven to 300 degrees. Coat the small baking dish with 2 tbsp of olive oil. Pour the red beans mixture in a baking dish and bake for about 10-15 minutes. You want to get a nice light brown color. Remove from the oven, let it stand for about 10 minutes and cut into 4 equal pieces. Serve warm.

Nutritional values per 100g:

Carbohydrates 26g

Sugar 12.5g

Protein 32.5 g

Total fat 7g

Sodium 612 mg

Potassium 84.1mg

Calcium 31mg

Iron 9mg

Vitamins (vitamin A; B-6; B-12; C; D; D2; D3; K; Riboflavin; Niacin; Thiamin; K)

Calories 179

43. Greek style chicken

Ingredients:

4 pieces of chicken breast halves

1 cup of cottage cheese

½ cup of Greek yogurt

1 cup of chopped cucumber

1 cup of chopped lettuce

1 cup of cherry tomatoes

½ cup of chopped onions

5 garlic cloves

2 tbsp of fresh lemon juice

1 tbsp of dried oregano

½ tsp of red pepper

½ tsp of salt

2 tbsp of olive oil

6 whole-wheat pitas, cut into wedges

Preparation:

Wash and cut the meat into small pieces. Set aside.

Combine the cottage cheese, Greek yogurt, vegetables and spices in a food processor. Mix well for 30 seconds. Heat up the olive oil over a medium temperature. Fry chicken chops for about 20 minutes, stirring constantly. Add the vegetable mixture to the saucepan. Stir well and cook for another 10 minutes. Remove from the heat and shape this mixture into 6 equal parts. Serve with pitas.

Nutritional values per 100g:

Carbohydrates 28.2g

Sugar 14.5g

Protein 33.5 g

Total fat 12g

Sodium 626.5 mg

Potassium 121.2mg

Calcium 34mg

Iron 10mg

Vitamins (vitamin A; B-6; B-12; C; D; D2; D3; K; Riboflavin; Niacin; Thiamin; K)

Calories 197

44. Lemon mushrooms

Ingredients:

4 thick chicken fillets

2 cups of button mushrooms, canned

1 cup of green beans, canned and cooked

1 1/3 cup of chicken broth

¼ cup of skim milk

1 tbsp of olive oil

¾ tsp of sea salt

½ tsp of ground black pepper

1 tsp of chopped fresh rosemary

4 tsp of all-purpose flour

2 tsp of fresh parsley, chopped

Preparation:

Wash and pat dry the chicken fillets. Preheat the oven to 300 degrees. Place green beans in a saucepan, cover with water and bring to a boil. Cook for about 10 minutes, or until tender. Remove from the heat and drain.

Combine salt, pepper, oil, skim milk and rosemary. Use a kitchen brush to spread this mixture over chicken. Place the chicken fillets at the bottom of a baking dish. Make another layer with green beans and button mushrooms. Combine chicken broth with flour and pour over chicken. Bake for about 35 minutes, until browned. Remove from the pan and sprinkle with fresh parsley. Serve warm.

Nutritional values per 100g:

Carbohydrates 29g

Sugar 12.1g

Protein 30.1 g

Total fat 11.9g

Sodium 522.1 mg

Potassium 104.9mg

Calcium 32mg

Iron 8.6mg

Vitamins (vitamin A; B-6; B-12; C; D; D2; D3; K; Riboflavin; Niacin; Thiamin; K)

Calories 157

45. Black bean tostadas

Ingredients:

1 cup of canned black beans, cooked

1 cup of red cabbage, finely chopped

2 pieces of chicken breast, shredded into large pieces

1 tbsp of chili sauce, sugar free

1 cup of low fat cream

½ tsp of salt

1 tsp of ground garlic

1 tsp of dry parsley

¼ tsp of ground black pepper

2 tbsp of fresh lemon juice

1 tbsp of brown sugar

1 tbsp of dry oregano

3 tbsp of olive oil

4 whole grain tortillas

Preparation:

Heat up the olive oil over medium-high temperature. First you want to fry tortillas, one at a time. They should be golden and crisp. This process will take 3-4 minutes for each tortilla. Soak the excess oil with kitchen paper.

Combine the beans and oregano and add to the saucepan. Stir well and fry for 2-3 minutes. Season with salt and pepper. Add garlic, parsley, lemon juice. Stir well and add chicken. Fry for about 20 minutes, stirring occasionally. Remove from the heat.

In a bowl, whisk together cabbage, low fat cream, chili sauce and sugar. You want a smooth and creamy mixture.

Top each tortilla with chicken mixture and cream dressing. Serve.

Nutritional values per 100g:

Carbohydrates 32.7g

Sugar 14g

Protein 34 g

Total fat 12.7g

Sodium 645 mg

Potassium 141.2mg

Calcium 23mg

Iron 7mg

Vitamins (vitamin A; B-6; B-12; C; D; D2; D3; K; Riboflavin; Niacin; Thiamin; K)

Calories 204

46. Orange barbecue

Ingredients:

4 large pieces of chicken breast, boneless

1 medium onion, chopped

2 small chili peppers

½ cup of chicken broth

¼ cup of fresh orange juice

1 tsp of orange extract

2 tbsp of olive oil

1 tsp of barbecue seasoning mix

1 cup of chopped lettuce

1 small red onion, chopped

Preparation:

Heat up the olive oil in a large saucepan. Add chopped onions and fry for several minutes, over a medium temperature – until golden color.

Combine chili peppers, orange juice and orange extract. Mix well in a food processor for 20-30 seconds. Add this mixture into a saucepan and stir well. Reduce heat to simmer.

Coat the chicken with barbecue seasoning mix and put into a saucepan. Add chicken broth and bring it to boil. Cook over a medium temperature until the water evaporates. Remove from the heat.

Serve with chopped lettuce and red onion.

Nutritional values per 100g:

Carbohydrates 26g

Sugar 11g

Protein 28.3 g

Total fat 9g

Sodium 421.1 mg

Potassium 128.1mg

Calcium 19mg

Iron 8.7mg

Vitamins (vitamin A; B-6; B-12; C; D; D2; D3; K; Riboflavin; Niacin; Thiamin; K)

Calories 186

47. Buffalo panini

Ingredients:

1 pound of chopped turkey breast

½ cup of Greek yogurt

½ cup of blue cheese

½ cup of cottage cheese

3 egg whites

1 tsp of curry sauce, sugar-free

1 tsp of almond butter

1 tsp of apple vinegar

1 tbsp of dried parsley

cooking spray

8 whole grain bread slices

Preparation:

In a large bowl, combine Greek yogurt with blue cheese, cottage cheese and egg whites. Mash well with a fork. You want a smooth mixture. Add curry sauce and vinegar. Mix well.

Sprinkle some cooking spray on a large saucepan. Heat up over a medium temperature. Add chopped turkey and fry for about 10 minutes, stirring constantly. Now add the cheese mixture, almond butter and dried parsley. Cook for about 5 minutes, until the cheese melts. Remove from the heat.

Spread this mixture over bread slices and serve.

Nutritional values per 100g:

Carbohydrates 29.2g

Sugar 16.1g

Protein 32.2 g

Total fat 10g

Sodium 611.4 mg

Potassium 102mg

Calcium 22mg

Iron 5.7mg

Vitamins (vitamin A; B-6; B-12; C; D; D2; D3; K; Riboflavin; Niacin; Thiamin; K)

Calories 171

48. High protein mac and cheese

Ingredients:

1 pound of chicken breast, boneless

1 cup of cottage cheese

1 cup of button mushrooms, canned

1 cup of whole grain macaroni

1 tsp of sea salt

1 tsp of butter

1 tsp of vegetable oil

Preparation:

Pour 3 cups of water in a pot. Bring it to boil and add macaroni and salt. Boil macaroni for about 7 minutes. You can also use the package instructions to cook macaroni. Remove from heat and drain.

Wash and pat dry the chicken. Cut into small pieces. In a large saucepan, melt 1 tsp of butter and add 1 tsp of vegetable oil. Heat up and add chicken pieces. Fry for about 15 minutes over a medium temperature. Add cottage cheese and mushrooms. Stir well and allow it to cook for few more minutes. Remove from the heat and add macaroni. Cover and allow it to stand for few minutes. Serve warm.

Nutritional values per 100g:

Carbohydrates 28g

Sugar 10.5g

Protein 30.1 g

Total fat 9.9g

Sodium 611.3 mg

Potassium 103 mg

Calcium 19mg

Iron 7.6mg

Vitamins (vitamin A; B-6; B-12; C; D; D2; D3; K; Riboflavin; Niacin; Thiamin; K)

Calories 177

OTHER GREAT TITLES BY THIS AUTHOR

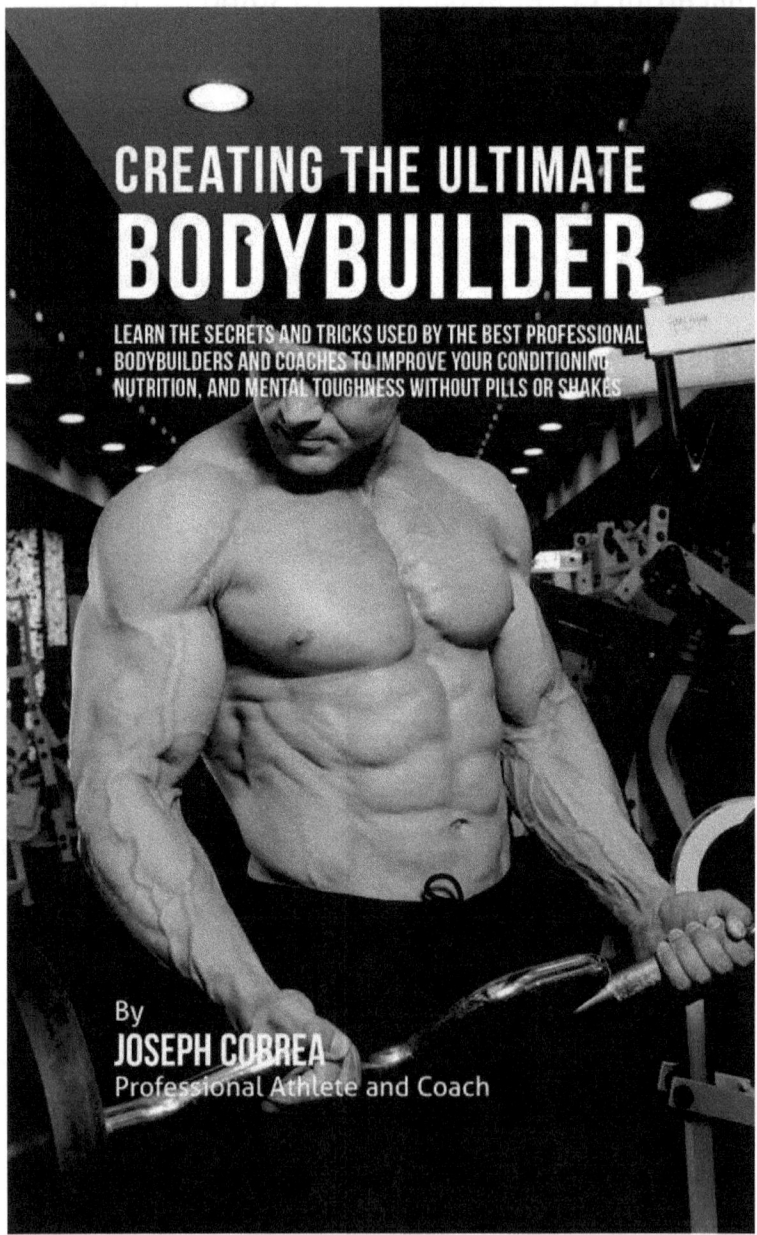

www.ingramcontent.com/pod-product-compliance
Lightning Source LLC
Chambersburg PA
CBHW071720020426
42333CB00017B/2344